ISBN 978-0-282-68704-5
PIBN 10861606

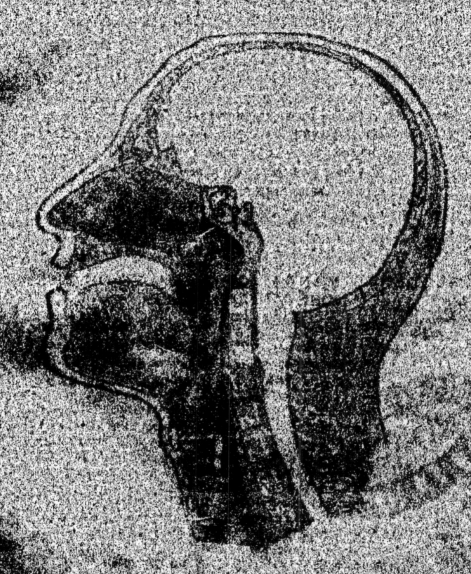

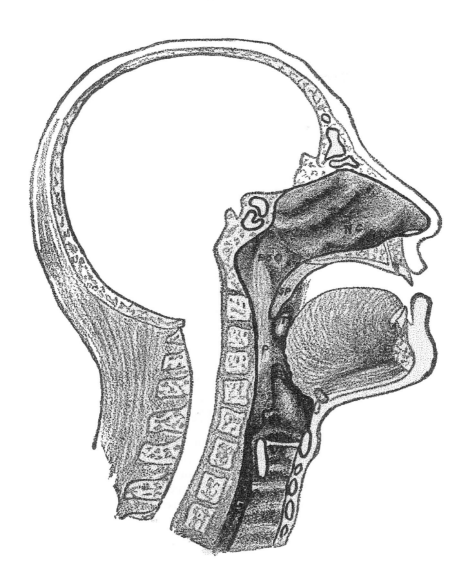

Medium cut of the head, showing the UPPER AIR TRACT in heavy outlines. NC, Nasal cavities and turbinated bones; EO, Eustachian orifice in the vault of the pharynx; SP, Soft palate and uvula; T, Left tonsil; P, Lower pharynx; E, Epiglottis; VB, Vocal band in the larynx; G, Œsophagus or gullet, the food passage.

CATARRH, SORE-THROAT

AND

HOARSENESS

A DESCRIPTION OF THE CONSTRUCTION, ACTION, AND USES
OF THE NASAL PASSAGES AND THROAT ; CERTAIN
DISEASES TO WHICH THEY ARE SUBJECT,
AND THE BEST METHODS FOR THEIR
PREVENTION AND CURE

BY

J. M. W. KITCHEN, M. D.

Assistant Surgeon to the Metropolitan Throat Hospital ; late Instructor
in Diseases of the Nose and Throat at the New York Post-
Graduate Medical School ; Assistant Physician to the
Bellevue Chest Class (O. D Dept.); Author of
"Students' Manual of Diseases of the
Nose and Throat"

————

G. P. PUTNAM'S SONS

NEW YORK : 27 & 29 WEST 23D STREET

COPYRIGHT BY
J. M. W. KITCHEN, M. D.
1884

Press of
G. P. Putnam'. Sons
New York

CONTENTS.

INTRODUCTORY.

CATARRH, SORE-THROAT, AND HOARSE-NESS are symptoms of disease in the nose, pharynx, and larynx, respectively. It is an undoubted fact that vast numbers of the human race suffer from the disorders producing these symptoms. It is computed that, in the United States, five millions of the inhabitants are more or less troubled with so-called catarrh. That the sufferers are multitudinous in number may be inferred when one takes note of the great number of nostrums that are advertised from year to year as " catarrh cures." Each of these preparations is, of course, the best and only cure for catarrh. The careful reader will often see advertised, certificates of cures following the use of these quack remedies. The failures to cure are not published. The surgeon meets many of these uncured cases at the hospital dispensary and in private practice. It is quite possible to formulate a catarrh cure that will meet the needs of a certain number of cases ; but that very formula will positively injure many other cases, and in any case requires intelligent application to be most effective.

It is hoped that a moderate attention to the subject-matter contained in the following pages will show the reader that catarrh is but a symptom of a variety of different diseased conditions, and that each condition requires its own peculiar, appropriate treatment for its cure. No single case is entirely like another, and even the same case may require widely varying methods of treatment at different stages of the disease. It is therefore impossible to devise a specific catarrh cure, and, to say the least, it is very unwise for a patient to experiment upon himself by using the proprietary remedies so widely advertised.

Within a comparatively few years there has been created in medical science a new branch known as LARYNGOLOGY, and with the scientific advancement of positive knowledge in this branch has grown up a set of practitioners who make a special study and practice of diseases of the nose and throat. Every practitioner of medicine should have taken a special course of instruction in diseases of the nose and throat, and should be able to treat any of the ordinary forms of disease that are met with in those organs ; but there are many cases that require the attention of the expert surgeon, who of necessity has to give years of study to, and to keep in constant active practice in, this special branch, to be able to afford satisfactory results in treatment. Intelligent and competent medical men, who have made a special study of these disorders, are now located in nearly all our large cities, and each year witnesses new acquisitions to the ranks of these specialists.

Probably in no other branch of medical science has such advance been made during the last few years in improved methods of treatment. It is therefore evident that sufferers from disease in these special organs need not, for their alleviation or cure, put their trust in the claims and promises

of advertising charlatans, as their troubles
can receive the intelligent attention of
trained specialists either in private practice or, if poverty prevents, in the dispensary practice of the throat departments now
established in connection with almost all
hospitals and dispensaries. It may be ad-
mitted that the ideas of the average layman
as to the nature of the disorders treated of
in this little book are decidedly misty. It
shall be the object of the writer in the following pages to endeavor to throw a little
light into this obscurity.

THE ANATOMICAL CONSTRUCTION AND HEALTHY ACTION OF THE NASAL PASSAGES AND THROAT.

IN order that the reader may gain any intelligent grasp of the subject, it is necessary that he should know something of the ANATOMY and PHYSIOLOGY of the parts where the morbid processes under discussion occur. These parts are the NASAL PASSAGES, PHARYNX, and LARYNX, a part of the human body often known as the UPPER AIR-TRACT, the lower continuation of which, connecting with the larynx, is composed of the trachea, bronchial tubes, and the final air-cells in the lung substance. (See fig. 1.)

All these parts form a continuous air-conduit from the external atmosphere to the net-work of minute blood-vessels surrounding the exceedingly thin membrane lining the air-cells. Through this thin lining the oxygen of the air is absorbed into the blood, and the surplus of carbonic-acid gas in the blood is given out to the air in the air-cells, and is from thence expired into the outer atmosphere by way of this same air-tract above mentioned.

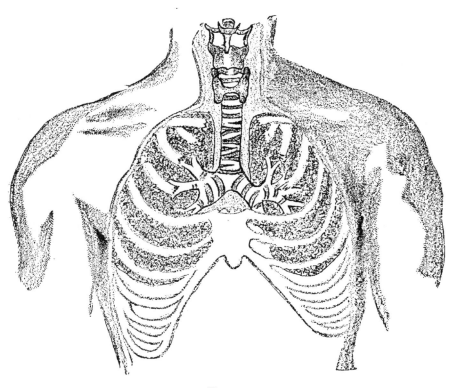

Fig. 1.

Representation of the larynx, trachea, bronchial tubes, and lungs in their relative positions in the body.

In the frontispiece the heavy dark lines indicate the outline of the upper air-tract, and the various parts important to our subject are named.   From the number of these named parts it may be rightly inferred that this part of the human body is not simply an air-tube, but that it is a rather complex machine, and has complex functions to fulfil.

What are these functions, and how are the organs formed for the fulfilling of their purpose?

I. THE NOSE is not only an air-passage, but it is arranged so as to detain on its sinuous surfaces, and by means of the hairs found inside the nostrils, a great deal of atmospheric dust and other impurities that would be likely to injure the delicate structure of the air-tract farther along. Its surfaces warm the passing air about two degrees F, and moisten it very considerably. The nose is also the organ of smell, and takes part in the formation and modification of articulate speech and song. The nasal passages are two irregularly triangular-shaped cavities, opening to the outer air by the two nostrils, and into the upper part of the pharynx by two oval-shaped openings known as the posterior nares. The walls of these cavities are of

bone at the back part, but the parts in
front of the plane of the face are mostly of
elastic cartilage, a provision very desirable
and convenient. Imagine the inconven-
ience of blowing or cleaning the nose if
the end of that organ was rigidly stiff, and
also consider the effect of the many bumps
and blows that seem a part of every child's
experience, upon so prominent a projection, if it was non-elastic. This elasticity
allows of considerable dilatation of the
nostrils, which movement is the result of
contraction in the neighboring small
muscles during the act of inspiration. The
two nasal passages are separated by a
partition known as the septum; this is
usually not quite straight, and when very
greatly bent the deviation is a cause of
disease. The outer surfaces of the bony
walls are much expanded in extent by their
structure. Three convolutions of bone extend out into the passages, and in the
mucous membrane covering these expanded surfaces are embedded the end filaments
of the special nerve of smell. These pro-
jections (see B. B., fig. 2.) are called the

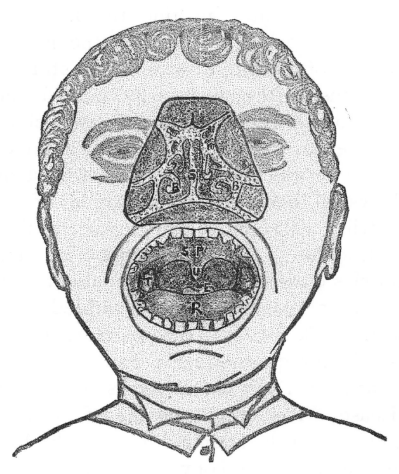

turbinated bones, and they fill about all of the space in the nasal passages that is not needed for the passage of air.

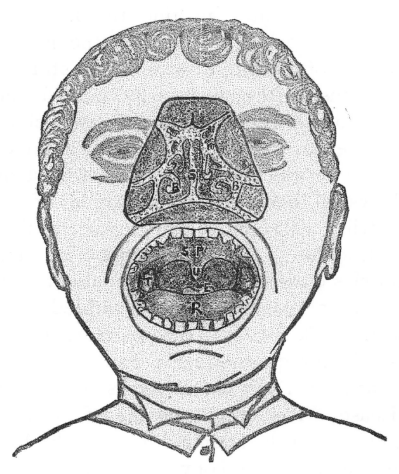

Fig. 2.

Transverse representation of the bony walls of the nose. B. B., Turbinated bones. S., Septum of the nose. Through the open mouth are seen the soft palate, S. P. The uvula, U. The right tonsil, T. The upper edge of the epiglottis, E. The tongue, R. The lower pharynx is at the back between the soft palate and the tongue.

Odoriferous particles are deposited on

these surfaces as air is drawn through the passages, and these produce that peculiar effect on the nerve filaments, which, being conveyed to the brain, gives to the individual the sensation known as smell. Mention must be made of several passages and cavities contiguous to and communicating with the nasal passages. These are, the lachrymal or tear-duct, which conveys the tears from the eye to the nose ; the frontal, maxillary, sphenoid, and ethmoid sinuses, which are located in the bones that compose the walls of the passages. They are apt to become diseased in conjunction with the nasal tract, and present difficult problems in the way of curative treatment on account of the difficulty in reaching the seat of trouble. These nasal passages and contiguous cavities have the further function of acting as resounding chambers in producing certain modifications and changes in the sounds of the voice, as will be explained further along.

II. THE PHARYNX acts as an air-passage, a resounding cavity for the voice, and the lower part of it as a food conveyer. It will be noticed by glancing at the frontispiece that in the lower part of the pharynx the air-tract and the food-tract cross each other, the food starting at the lips and being carried to the stomach by way of the mouth, lower pharynx, and the œsophagus or gullet. The mouth is also an accessory air-tract brought into use during unusual exertion and consequent need of an increased air supply, but the normal healthy method of breathing is through the nose with the mouth shut. The pharynx extends from the base of the brain to, and is continuous with, the œsophagus. The soft palate is a flexible curtain, which is the continuation backward and downward of the hard roof of the mouth. It has mucous membrane on both of its sides, enclosing muscles that will contract and draw it upward and backward.

When these muscles are relaxed, the soft palate hangs downward, and in the middle line of its lower edge will be seen a short dependent projection known as the uvula (see U. fig 2). In this state of relaxation there is a free passage for air from the mouth to the nasal passages, and all parts of the pharynx constitute one continuous tract; but when the soft palate is contracted and raised upward and backward, it divides the pharynx into two parts, which may be called the vault of the pharynx, and the lower pharynx. The latter opens into the mouth, and is the part seen when looking directly backward through the open mouth. The posterior apertures of the nasal passages open directly into the vault of the pharynx, and this latter place should properly be considered as a part of the nasal passages. It is a sort of retired corner in the air-tract, and dust and the secretions of its mucous membrane are apt to become lodged there, acting as an irritant to the parts.

The lower pharynx has the advantage over the vault, in that its surfaces are swept, and thus cleansed, by every mouthful of food swallowed. The unclean condition of the pharyngeal vault acts as a cause in bringing about and keeping up the disease known as post-nasal catarrh, the most common disease of this part of the body

that falls to the care of the medical practitioner. In the sides of this vault are located the orifices of the Eustachian tubes,
two passages that convey air into the middle ears. Inflammation of this part of the
air-tract is apt to extend along these tubes,
producing ear-troubles. Indeed, simple
stoppage of the orifices of these tubes from
an excess of mucus secreted in the back
part of the nose or upper part of the
pharynx may more or less interfere with
the function of hearing. In examining the
lower pharynx, we find at the base of the
tongue, leading forward and downward
from the pharynx, the opening into the
larynx or beginning of the windpipe proper, which latter tube runs perpendicularly
down the neck in front of the œsophagus.
The œsophagus is always relaxed and flat-
tened out, except when food is passing
through it, while the windpipe is always
kept open by stiff, cartilaginous, nearly
complete rings which fulfil that purpose.
Leading from the soft palate on each side,
downward to the tongue, are two folds of
mucous membrane known as the pillars of

the fauces, and between them are the organs known as the tonsils. These glands are much subject to inflammation and to inflammatory changes. They are two almond-shaped bodies composed of bunched folds of mucous membrane, and are abundantly furnished with glands which produce a viscid mucous secretion useful for lubricating the parts, thus facilitating the passage of food during the act of swallowing. This act of swallowing is brought about through the agency of muscular bands which surround the back of the pharynx, and which act involuntarily in grasping any bolus of food that has been pressed far enough back by the tongue, and in pressing the food downward into the œsophagus, where the contraction of successive layers of muscles press the bolus along into the stomach. It will be observed that the food has to pass directly over the opening into the larynx, and on this account the top of the larynx closes tightly during every act of swallowing, and any attempt to draw air into the windpipe during the act, or of breathing through the mouth while food is in it, is apt to draw food into the larynx, causing the spasmodic cough that is noticed when food particles go "the wrong way." The act of swallowing necessitates a great deal of motion in the parts composing the pharynx, and on this account are felt the pain and discomfort that accompany inflammation in this locality. This is the part of the upper air-tract usually affected in ordinary so-called sore throats.

III. THE LARYNX has very complex functions to fulfil. It is an air-passage. It is also a valve that can close so tight that food cannot enter it, or air cannot escape when it is desirable to hold the lungs full of it; or it can be so regulated that the air may escape more or less freely as may be desired. This valve is opened during every inspiration by direct muscular exertion on the part of the muscles of the larynx, which relax during the ensuing expiration, unless the expiration is a restricted one. The larynx is supplied with the vocal apparatus that enables it to produce what is known as voice. This little machine which is so capable of producing an almost endless variety of sounds, pleasing or otherwise, is sometimes called a vocal box. It is walled in by several stiff, cartilaginous structures, all more or less movable, but together forming the frame-

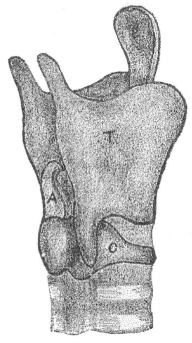

Fig. 3.

Cartilages of the larynx. E, epiglottis. A, left arytenoid cartilage. T, thyroid cartilage. C, cricoid cartilage resting on the trachea.

work of the larynx, preserving its shape and affording points of attachment for the various membranes, ligaments, muscles, etc., that constitute its make-up. These cartilages are represented in fig. 3.

There is at the top of the trachea a cartilaginous ring known as the cricoid cartilage, shaped somewhat like a seal-ring. Rocking on this, with the joint at the back, and connected with it at the sides and in front by a thin flexible membrane, is the large thyroid cartilage, a shield-shaped

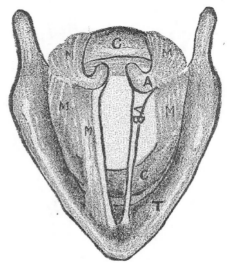

Fig. 4.

Interior view of the larynx, looking from above downward. VB, left vocal cord or band. T, thyroid cartilage. C, C, cricoid cartilage. A, apex of left arytenoid cartilage. M, M, M, M, M, muscles.

body whose projected front forms the prominence at the front of the neck, well known as "Adam's apple." At the back of the cricoid cartilage and resting on it are two pyramidal bodies known as the arytenoid cartilages. These partly revolve

on their bases, as if on pivots.   Attached
to and running between these cartilages
and the inner surface of the front of the
thyroid cartilage, are the two white fibrous
bands known as the vocal bands or cords
(see fig. 4).   These vocal bands, though
a part of the mucous membrane lining the

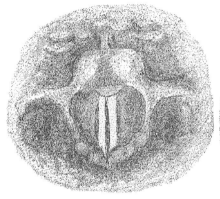 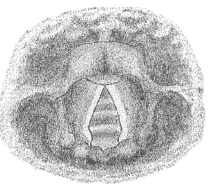

Fig. 5.

Interior of the larynx with
the vocal bands adducted or
approximated, the position
taken during phonation or
voice production.

Fig. 6.

Interior of the larynx with
the vocal bands drawn apart
or abducted, being the position
taken during inspiration. The
white rings of the trachea show
between the separated vocal
bands.

larynx, differ in structure, being of a white
fibrous material essentially the same as the
white tissue that forms in the cicatrix of a
wound.   To these various movable cartilages are attached muscles (some are seen
in fig. 4) which, when called into action,

can make these vocal bands more or less tense or flaccid, or can bring them together so that their edges are approximated, as in fig. 5, or can open them widely at the back part of the larynx, as in fig. 6. Indeed, at every inspiration taken, the muscles that open this aperture of the larynx or glottis, as it is often called, are brought into action, and it will thus be seen that there is incessant active motion in this organ. This is one reason why some laryngeal disorders are difficult to cure. Above the thyroid cartilage, in the folds of mucous membrane, are small muscles which help to press together the opening of the larynx when that action is necessary. Above all is the epiglottis, very much like the lid of a molasses jug, that can be pulled downward and backward over the opening of the larynx, allowing food and drink to slide over it into the œsophagus.

A word as to the mucous membrane lining this upper air-tract. The prominent purpose served by this structure is to furnish a mucous secretion that shall properly moisten and lubricate the parts, protecting them from injurious influences, such as the friction that would take place if the parts were dry, or from the immediate contact of dust, vapors, and other irritating substances. This protective action is always needed, for the ordinary atmospheric impurities, such as dust, plant-pollen, disease-germs, etc., settle continually on the slight layer of

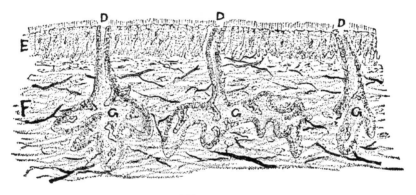

Fig. 7.

Schematic representation of the mucous membrane of the upper air-tract. E, epithelial cells of the surface of the membrane. F, deep layer of fibrous or elastic tissue containing the glands G, G, G, blood-vessels, nerves, etc. D, D, D, orifices to the ducts of the secreting glands.

mucus protecting the membrane, and is now and then ejected from the air-tract by means of blowing the nose, swallowing, or expectoration. Fig. 7 is a schematic representation of a part of the mucous membrane of the upper air-tract. It represents a section cut transversely from the surface to the

deeper layers, or to the bony wall. Among
the principal features to be noticed are the
mucous glands. These are compound in
structure, and each one has a duct leading
to the surface of the mucous membrane.
These glands are thickly placed in the mucous membrane, and are lined with small
cells which secrete the mucus that finds its
exit through the ducts to the surface. The
next feature to be observed is the cells that
form the surface of the mucous membrane.
These are narrow and oblong in shape, and
are furnished at their free edge with an
immense number of small tail-like projec-
tions known as ciliæ. These little ciliæ, in
the living mucous membrane, keep up a
continuous rapid, waving vibration, that,
under the microscope, looks like the waving
of a field of tall grain swept by a brisk
breeze. The object of this waving motion
is to convey from the air-tract the excreted
mucus and such foreign substances as dust,
etc., that may be lodged on it. The mucous membrane is also furnished with blood-
vessels and nerves, and the whole structure
is completed and held together with various

differing cells, and a fibrous elastic material known as connective tissue. In chronic inflammation this fibrous tissue is apt to increase in quantity, and subsequently contract, pressing out of existence those very important parts of the structure, the glands. This matter will be further spoken of in a · following chapter.

A general understanding of the method of voice production is necessary to comprehend the causes of hoarseness. If the edges of the vocal bands are brought by the appropriate muscles so that they are in apposition, as in fig. 5, and certain other muscles exert a pulling power at the ends of the bands, so that they are held in a certain degree of tension, and at the same time air is driven through the oblong slit between them, the vocal bands which are elastic, will be first pushed up somewhat and will then rebound. Then the outgoing air will push them up again, and so on. In short, they will vibrate. This vibration breaks the out-going column of air into waves, and these air-waves, striking the drum of the ear, cause it also to vibrate, and in turn communicate its motion to the delicate auditory apparatus in connection with the nerves in the ear. This impression being conveyed along the nerve-tract to the brain, will produce that sensation known as a voice-sound. This act of the larynx is known scientifically as *phonation.*

If the to-and-fro vibration of the vocal bands occurs about twenty-five times in one second there will be formed a very low

Fig. 8.   Fig. 9.

bass note. If the vibration be twenty-five hundred times in one second, there will be formed a very high treble note. These will be about the lowest and highest notes that can be formed by the human larynx. If this to-and-fro vibration of the vocal cord or band be very great, as is illustrated in fig. 8, the sound will be very loud. If, on the contrary, a mild, gentle sound issues from the larynx, we may know that the extent of the to-and-fro motion is small as in fig. 9.

The *pitch* of the sound, that is, the relative highness or lowness of the note in the musical scale, will depend upon the length and thickness of the vocal bands and the degree of tension to which they are subjected.   The tighter and shorter the vocal band, the higher its pitch will be, just as in the strings of a piano. · However, the sound-producer of the human larynx is not like the sound-producer of any one musical instrument, though it is somewhat like the vibrating reed of a reed instrument.   The important point for the reader to remember is, that this vocal apparatus is actuated by a number of muscles, and when in use it is subject to ever-varying motion, strain, and variety of position, and, consequently, a great deal of wear and tear.   The vibrating column of air, after its production in the larynx, reverberates through the other air-passages.   Some low tones reverberate in the air-passages below the larynx, and are known as chest tones.   Certain others, known as head tones, gain their quality by having their reverberations confined to the cavities above the larynx.   Other modulalations and variations of speech and song are the result of change of shape in the reverberatory passages, caused by the various positions taken by the mouth, soft palate, tongue, teeth, and lips, together with varying pressures of air from the lungs. Some of the sounds are the result of the vibrating air-column being sent through the nasal passages, others through the mouth alone, while still others are produced by the combined use of the two passages. It will be readily understood that the natural conformation of the parts concerned in voice production, as well as their health status, have a very direct relation to the quality of the voice and the healthy action of the voice-producing apparatus.

IN order that the Nasal Passages, Pharynx, and Larynx be maintained in a good state of health, it is necessary :

FIRST.—That the parts be well nourished by a blood-supply that shall contain the necessary elements of nutrition, and be free from those excessive impurities which result from imperfect elaboration, secretion, and excretion of the various important organs of the body, such as the stomach, liver, kidneys, etc. This implies the necessity of eating proper food, both in quality and quantity, and the living of a generally correct hygienic life on the part of the individual. Blood impurities that may interfere with the health of the parts under consideration, may be the result of diseased principles that have gained access to the body from without ; for example, the poisons of scarlet-fever and diphtheria, which produce certain symptoms of throat disease, represent impurities received from outside the body, while the irritant that produces gout represents an impurity that originates internally.

SECOND.—That all the parts be used sufficiently to develop their full functional activity, otherwise the tissues entering into their construction deteriorate and become unhealthy. The nasal passages are the normal routes for the passage of air, and the mouth is only an auxiliary avenue to be used in case of great exertion. If an individual habitually breathes through the mouth, the nasal structures miss the natural stimulus of the rush of air through them, and the result is a relaxed condition of the mucous membrane that leaves it in a state inviting attacks of disease. Furthermore, the air entering the mouth arrives at the throat cooler, dryer, and contaminated with more impurities than if it came through the nasal passages, and hence it is more irritating to the pharynx, and, in lesser measure, to the rest of the air-tract.

The voice should be regularly used, but yet not abused ; as, for example, by too long talking ; or strained by too loud phonation, as in shouting ; or by excessive tension, as in striking too highly pitched notes in singing, etc.   The voice can be much strengthened by judicious culture.   Reading aloud and singing may thus be made hygienic procedures, as well as agreeable pastimes.

THIRD.—That the air-passages should not be made delicate through *excessive* protection from the ordinary wear and tear and irritations of surrounding atmospheric influences, such as temperature-changes, etc. The pursuit of the ordinary avocations of life requires that this part of the body be exposed to a certain amount of these influences, and that they should not produce a deleterious effect, it is necessary to somewhat accustom the air-tract to exposure to stimulative irritation, but this exposure should not be overdone. When the breathing of very cold air is a necessity for a part of the day, the individual should be careful not to breathe for any length of time an overheated atmosphere in the house, espe-

cially during the sleeping hours, which atmosphere would tend to weaken the mucous membrane lining the air-passages, and
make it more sensitive to the deleterious
influences of the very cold out-of-door air.
The breathing of impure air should be
avoided, as it will not only irritate the air-
passages, but will produce a depressing effect upon the general health. The throat
should not be weakened by over-clothing
the neck. Clothing should be equably dis-
tributed over the body. When a large fur
collar is worn around the neck that part is
overheated and weakened. Enough clothing, but no more, should be worn to keep
the body up to the normal healthy temperature of 98°, and the clothing should be
regulated as to quantity in strict reference to the amount of exposure of the individual to cold, winds, moisture, etc.
One of the best methods of becoming
accustomed to the effect of undue exposure
to cold, is to adopt the practice of sponging
the body with cold water, and to follow
this by a brisk rubbing until reaction occurs, producing a fine glow in the skin.

This practice, besides being a good general tonic and stimulant, toughens the skin, and renders it less sensitive to temperature changes.

FOURTH.—That undue exposure be avoided to such causes as would provoke disease in the parts, as, for example, excessive high or low temperatures. Air should not be breathed that is laden with such irritating dust vapors or gases as may prove prejudicial to the good-health status of the parts under discussion. Where exposures to such irritants are unavoidable, the wearing of a respirator will be very desirable in preventing the usual troublesome results. There are various good respirators sold by the instrument-makers, but a home-manufactured article answers every purpose. A bunch of thin gauzy fabric, such as ladies use for veils, held or fastened over the nose and mouth, is sufficient. This will act mechanically to strain from the air many of its atmospheric impurities; and the expired air, being somewhat retained in the meshes of the material, warms the ingoing air very considerably, which thus loses in a measure its injurious influences. Where a tendency exists to affections of the air-passages, the adoption of the open-grate fire, as a means of heating and ventilation, is almost a necessity in the prevention, and in the curative treatment, of diseases of these parts. This method of heating gives ample opportunity to warm the body just to the degree of its requirements by direct radiation, without overheating the air respired. It gives a fine mechanical ventilation to the apartment in which it is located, and in the removals of the body to and from the fire one is subject to such frequent changes of temperature that the formation of a delicate habit is prevented, and the individual is inured in a measure to the temperature-changes that must be met in the best-protected life.

ON CERTAIN DISEASED CONDITIONS AND PROCESSES TO WHICH THE PARTS ARE SUBJECT.

THE mucous membrane, as well as the deeper structures entering into the construction of the upper air-tract, may exhibit a departure from the healthy state in many ways. Among others—the parts may be too poorly nourished. They may be in a state of excessive nourishment. They may be inflamed. There may be a loss of function or usefulness in the parts. There may be excessive functional activity. There may be diseased growths present.

FIRST.—With regard to a poor state of nutrition. In this condition the parts are relaxed and lack tone. They are not able to meet the wear and tear of the ordinary uses required of them. They are more liable to attacks of the more serious diseased processes. This condition may be the result of a poor state of nutrition of the whole body, or it may be due to lack of use of the parts, or, in other words, of calling out their functional activity. For example, if a person breathes habitually through the mouth, the nasal passages will be apt to fall into this condition. Ulcerations or loss of tissue are liable to be present in this state.

SECOND.—The state of over-nourishment is one in which there is too great an amount of blood supplied to the parts, which 'are swollen and red, and in an irritable, sensitive state too easily aggravated into more serious conditions by even the ordinary atmospheric influences present, as well as through the ordinary use of the parts. This condition is apt to be present in those who use alcoholic beverages ; the alcohol acting either as a direct irritant to the parts while being swallowed, or by increasing the force of the general circulation, or in other ways in furnishing too great a local blood-supply.

THIRD.—Inflammation is a difficult thing to define even to the professional student. We can only say that it is a process marked by certain phenomena. These are mainly, an increased blood-supply to, and elevation of temperature in, the part inflamed, with more rapid waste in the diseased tissue. The increase of temperature may extend to the whole body. There is swelling and pain, and if the process progresses to a certain extent, the formation of pus, and perhaps even the production of gangrene or death of the part will take place. If the part inflamed be a mucous membrane, as in the nose, pharynx, and larynx, the production of the mucous secretion will be interfered with ; at first there will be a deficiency, but later on there will be a greater production than is natural. There is also apt to be an extensive increase in the shedding of the cells that compose the surface of the mucous membrane. If the inflammation be deep, the pus formed collects in a cavity forming an abscess, from which after a certain maturity, the pus works its way to the surface, and, with a free vent thus formed, the process usually comes to an end. This is the process that occurs in the familiar throat trouble known as Quinsy sore-throat. In the mucous membrane, as a rule, the pus finds its way to the surface without forming in collections or abscesses. If muscles are involved in the inflammatory process their action will be interfered with so as to produce more or less paralysis in them. If the process goes through a regular course in a few days, or a week or so, it is called an acute inflammation, and after the parts become quieted down to their normal state it will be found that no considerable changes have occurred in the parts themselves. Chronic inflammation extends over weeks and even years, and is not characterized by such severity of action as the acute attack ; but, if it persists a certain time there will be changes of a decided nature in the anatomical elements forming the structure of the parts inflamed. There may be an increase in all the elements, or some one element may preponderate in the increase. Take, for instance, a chronic inflammation of the mucous membrane of the pharynx ; the glands may be the element mostly affected, and become much enlarged, producing the condition known as Clergyman's sore-throat. As another example : in a chronic inflammation of the mucous membrane of the nose, the fibrous element in the membrane may become increased and afterward contract, completely obliterating the glands, thus producing ozæna or fetid catarrh, that very unfortunate complaint, hard to endure both by the patient and those with whom he is brought in contact. It is of course only attempted here to outline something of the nature of these diseased processes. A complete idea of the nature of inflammation requires years of study for its comprehension.

FOURTH.—There may be loss of function in a part. Among the conditions coming under this head, may be loss or impairment of the voice, such as hoarseness ; difficulty in swallowing, or in the articulating powers ; loss of smell, etc. These disorders may be caused primarily by some diseased condition of the parts themselves, or they may be secondary to some trouble either in the parts themselves, or in some distant locality, as in the nervous system.

Many of these affections may be classed under the head of paralysis, and this paralysis may be due to inflammation, presence of growths, hysteria, etc.

FIFTH.—Excessive functional activity in the upper air-tract is chiefly noticeable in the production of excessive secretion by the glands. Frequently the muscular apparatus of the throat is implicated, having an involuntary action of a spasmodic nature, an example of which is so often seen in the so-called spasmodic croup. Other examples, are where excessive sensibility of the sense of smell and great irritability of some part of the mucous membrane exist. An hysterical tendency in an individual will tend to develop these diseased peculiarities.

SIXTH.—There are various kinds of growths that occur in the nasal passages, pharynx, and larynx. Some are so benign that they may not materially interfere with the usefulness of the organs invaded. Others are not dangerous to life, and can be removed without permanent injury to the individual, while still others are but manifestations in the upper air-tract of serious if not absolutely fatal disease that involves more or less of the whole body. As examples of the latter may be mentioned malignant cancer, and tuberculosis or consumption of the larynx. In the very serious cases, the diseased growths in forming displace and destroy the natural healthy parts, and then finally break down themselves, ulcerating and leaving vast cavities. In some of the serious cases the ravages of the disease may be stopped and life saved, but after healing the parts are left permanently deformed.

All the above conditions and processes, and others not mentioned, may either be present in connection with, or have been the cause in the production of, one or other of the symptoms known as Catarrh, Sore-Throat, and Hoarseness.

ACUTE Nasal Catarrh, or Cold in
the Head, or Coryza.—This is a
transient inflammation of the mucous
membrane of the nasal cavities, the contiguous cavities being usually affected
also. It is marked by swelling and
stuffiness in the nose, followed by a discharge, at first thin and watery, but which
later becomes thick. The attack usually
passes off, in from three to ten days, spon-
taneously. It can sometimes be aborted,
and can always be much shortened in its
duration, and alleviated by appropriate
local treatment.

Chronic Nasal Catarrh is characterized by a persistent abnormal discharge
from the nose. There are various conditions that may be present in this disorder. The discharge may be thin, watery,

and abundant, or it may be scanty and tenacious, and fetid in odor. The mucous membrane may be thickened, or in other cases it may be atrophied or shrunken away. This condition requires long and varying treatment, and in some cases surgical operations, to bring about a cure.

OBSTRUCTION OF THE NASAL PASSAGES FROM GROWTHS AND MALFORMATIONS may become a cause of disease, as well as a disease itself. Surgical procedures are generally necessary for its correction.

FETID NASAL CATARRH, sometimes known as Dry Catarrh or Ozæna, is a most unfortunate disorder for the possessor and all those with whom he is brought in contact. The terrible stench emanating from the nostrils repels even the warmest friend. If this affection has continued too long, it is not possible to entirely cure the case, but every case can be much improved, and the patient can be brought into such a condition that his life will not be a burden, and he will cease to be a nuisance to his friends. Some cases are entirely curable.

ULCERATIONS IN THE NOSE are sores

that do not heal, and that result in the loss of tissue. They may be the result of a poorly nourished condition of the parts, and readity heal under an appropriate stimulating treatment; but the great cause of this condition is the ravages of syphilis, that terrible venereal disease that is the scourge of the world. If not promptly checked by the most energetic medical measures, there may be much destruction in the parts, resulting in great permanent deformity.

HAY FEVER is a disease of which the peculiar characteristic is a profuse watery catarrh from the nasal passages. It can be much alleviated by suitable medicated applications, but cure can only be assured by the removal of the patient to a locality where the atmosphere is free from the irritating plant pollen, etc., which is the cause of the disease.

FOREIGN BODIES IN THE NOSE, which have become impacted in the sinuosities of the nasal passages by children, generally too young to know of their wrong-doing, usually set up a persistent, though slight catarrh. There may be a slow inflammatory action present that eventually will enlarge the tissues and shut in the body from view, but a thorough examination by the surgeon will generally discover the cause of trouble, and the removal of the body brings about a cure.

ACUTE SORE-THROAT—Almost everybody has experienced this trouble. It is a transient inflammation of the mucous membrane of the lower pharynx and neighboring parts, and its chief symptom is a painful sensation occurring during the act of swallowing. It is usually self-limited to a very few days' duration. If taken at the start it may usually be cured in one, or at least two days, by skilful treatment. This is one of the few throat complaints that can be successfully treated by the patient at home. (See Chapter on Domestic Treatment.)

CHRONIC SORE-THROAT, often called Clergyman's Sore-Throat, is the result of a long course of abuse of the pharynx. The changes in the mucous membrane are marked, especially in the glands, which become enlarged. The curative treatment is generally very tedious, and in some cases rather severe measures have to be adopted to bring about a change for the better.

POST-NASAL CATARRH is the name of a catarrhal affection of the vault of the pharynx, generally chronic in character and associated with nasal catarrh. It is *the* throat and nasal affection most frequently treated by the professional man, and is exceedingly common. Its treatment requires much attention at home by the patient, in the way of constant cleansing, as it occurs just at the remote angle in the air-tract, where impurities, such as dust, together with the abnormal secretions, are apt to become lodged, and further provoke diseased action in the part.

INFLAMMATION OF THE TONSILS.—Some people have a predisposition to inflammation of these glands. The inflammation may only implicate the surface of the tonsils and their deep folds or follicles, which trouble is often mistaken for diphtheria by ignorant practitioners, and, being so designated by them, these men get the reputation for effecting great cures.

QUINSY SORE-THROAT is a deep inflammation of the tonsils in which there is formed one or more abscesses. It is an exceedingly painful and severe disorder, causing great general prostration, and almost closing the mouth, so that swallowing or even opening the mouth is extremely difficult. Children and young people who have these attacks of tonsillar trouble are apt to have their tonsils become permanently enlarged. All of these cases are much improved by the removal of the enlarged organs. In some cases their removal is imperatively necessary, as they interfere with breathing, and thus lead to a deformity of the chest that causes future trouble in the lungs. These enlarged glands may interfere with the hearing, with proper articulation in speech, and with the general nutrition, on account of the difficulty they cause in swallowing.

A RELAXED SOFT PALATE AND ELONGATED UVULA may cause a persistent inflammatory condition, not only of the pharynx, but of the larynx as well. The trouble may usually be rectified by simple applications of astringents and stimulants, but frequently the removal of a portion of the uvula is a necessity. It is not a painful operation, and affords great relief.

DIPHTHERIA, though a septic disease of the whole body, may be mentioned here, because it peculiarly manifests itself in an intense inflammation of the throat. Sometimes its only manifestation is a slight sore-throat. These slight sore-throats are apt to be present during epidemics of diphtheria. This disease is apt to leave the muscles of the throat in a paralyzed condition, thus becoming one cause of hoarseness and difficulty in swallowing. Of course this dangerous disease requires the immediate and constant care of a trained physician.

ULCERATED SORE-THROAT may be due to a poorly nourished condition, or to a pecullar inflammatory state ; but usually it is the result of syphilitic formations in the tissues of the throat, and these, breaking down, produce the ulcerated condition.

CROUP is the designation given by the laity to almost every acute affection of the larynx. There are a number of inflammatory and functional disorders that are so called, but whatever the affection may be, the prominent feature which arrests the attention, is the impairment of the voice known as hoarseness. The exception to this is the affection known as spasmodic croup, when uncomplicated with inflammation ; in which case the difficulty in breathing, and the hard, brassy, croupy cough, are the prominent signs. This latter trouble is simply a spasm of the muscles of the larynx, and comes as a reflex action from some distant source of irritation, as, for example, the presence of an excess of indigestible matter in the alimentary canal. Though alarming, this condition is not a serious one, but when it occurs in connection with an acute catarrhal inflammation of the larynx, it is a serious disorder, and needs the prompt attention of an intelligent physician. In children these inflammatory laryngeal troubles are serious, because the swelling of the mucous membrane encroaches so much upon the naturally small air-space in the larynx, all of which is needed for the passage of air. In some of these cases an immediate artificial opening into the windpipe, through the front of the neck, is imperatively necessary to save the life of the patient. The ordinary mild attacks of "croup," or acute catarrhal laryngitis, in the adult, usually result in self-cure in the course of a week or ten days, if the patient be only careful to avoid exposures to any cause that would increase the difficulty by further irritation ; but proper medicinal local applications to the larynx by the surgeon will afford great relief and materially shorten the duration of the attack. If the inflammation be very severe, or is the result of diphtheria, there is apt to form in the larynx a false membrane that may fill up the air-space so that more or less speedy suffocation of the patient ensues. These cases usually end fatally, though a few do recover.

CHRONIC LARYNGITIS may, among other causes, be the result of a neglected acute inflammatory attack, or it may be due to a long-continued irritation, as from over use of the larynx. The mucous membrane becomes unequally thickened and other-

wise changed. Though there will be disagreeable symptoms, such as burning,
tickling, excessive secretion, cough, etc.,
the prominent symptom is apt to be some
impairment of the voice. Either there will
be hoarseness, or the voice cannot be con-
trolled as well as usual ; a condition more
noticeable in singing and declamation.
Some of these cases merely require rest of
the voice to bring about a cure, but the
great majority require local medicinal applications in the larynx. Some of these cases
prove to be very obstinate, and require
great perseverance on the part of the
patient in submitting to continued treatment before a cure can be effected. Some
very bad cases of long standing can only
be promised alleviation and improvement.
It is most important, if these patients ex-
pect to be cured, that they do not neglect
early treatment, and they should not allow
the trouble to exist for any length of time
without consulting a trained physician.

PARALYSIS OF THE LARYNGEAL MUSCLES
may cause hoarseness, and even loss of
voice or *aphonia*. The condition may be

a temporary one, caused, for instance, by an acute inflammation, and resulting in self-cure upon subsidence of the inflammatory attack. Other cases may be amenable to treatment, and especially to applications of electricity. Still other cases are absolutely incurable, and if certain muscles are affected, the result is apt to be fatal.

CANCER, CONSUMPTION, AND SYPHILIS OF THE LARYNX are all troubles, fortunately not very common, whose first symptom may be hoarseness of the voice. The first two are almost always fatal in the end. The diseases here mentioned are only among those that are commonly met with, having a connection with our subject. Enough, however, have been cited, to show how great a variety of disorders may be the cause of the symptoms known as CATARRH, SORE-THROAT, AND HOARSENESS.

CERTAIN SYMPTOMS OF NASAL AND THROAT DISORDERS AND THEIR SIGNIFICANCE.

BAD BREATH is caused by vitiation or putrefaction of the secretions of the food- and air-tracts. It may also result from putrefaction of broken-down tissues of those parts, as in ulcerative processes. It may come from imperfect or unclean teeth, disordered stomach, fermenting food, ulcerating growths, decomposing secretion in the follicles of the tonsils, and retained secretion in the bronchial tubes. One of the most terribly offensive breaths is the result of dry catarrh in the nose, and also that produced by large masses of retained and putrefying secretions in the cavities adjoining and emptying into the nose. Deep ulcerations in the nose, producing cavities containing decomposing broken-down tissue, give rise to an indescribably terrible stench.

CATARRH.—The ideas of the average layman on the nature of catarrh are not only vague, but usually incorrect. Scientifically the word signifies an inflammatory discharge of fluid from any mucous membrane in the body, but ˙the word, in common parlance, is used to designate an abnormal discharge from the nasal cavities and from the vault of the pharynx. The ancients thought that this discharge was an efflux from the brain, discharging certain morbid humors from the system. Even in this later day of supposed enlightenment, quacks and charlatans, who advertise catarrhal remedies, claim that a catarrhal discharge is the result of the presence of these vicious humors in the blood, which find vent from the nose. Of course, their pet remedy will search out and eliminate all such disagreeable constituents of the nourishing fluid. The glands of the air-tract normally discharge a certain amount of secretion, whose purpose is to keep the parts properly moistened and lubricated. A catarrhal discharge may merely be an excessive production of this secretion, and this simply indicates an over-stimulation of the glands from some cause. If the secretion is very thin and watery, it is due to a large amount of the serum of the blood being exuded from the mucous membrane. This is present in the first part of acute catarrhal discharges. In proportion as this watery serum is wanting, the discharge becomes thick and more sticky, owing to a greater proportionate amount of mucus being present. In violent inflammation, and in the later stages of milder ones, the discharge becomes clouded, owing to the presence of pus-cells, and also to the shedding of many of the small cells composing the outer layer of the mucous membrane. If there are ulcerations present, the discharge may be colored with blood. A nasal catarrh may be the result of an acute inflammation or a chronic one. It may be confined to the nasal passages, or the connecting cavities may also be implicated. It may be the result of ulcerations in the nose, or be due to the presence of a foreign body, or of growths in the nose.

Cough, when caused by inflammatory

tickling or presence of secretion in the larynx, has a peculiar brassy tone known as a " croupy cough." There is also a peculiar cough used to expel secretion from the lower pharynx.

DIFFICULTY IN SWALLOWING. — This symptom may be the result of paralysis of the muscles used in the act, or it may be due to a swollen condition of any of the parts of the throat. It may also be caused by growths, especially those in the lower part of the pharynx, obstructing the passage of food. Spasm of the pharyngeal muscles will also make swallowing difficult.

DRYNESS AND BURNING in the throat may be due to deficient secretion, or may be one of the sensations of the inflammatory process.

EXPECTORATION. — Children under six years of age, as a rule, do not expectorate. Expectorated matter usually comes from the lower pharynx, larynx, or bronchial tubes, but it is frequently the secretion of the mucous membrane back of the nose, which reaches the mouth by dropping into it, or by being drawn backward and downward by an inspiratory effort.

HAWKING is the act of clearing the pharynx from excessive or redundant secretions. It is usually caused by morbid secretions being formed at the back of the nasal passages and in the vault of the pharynx, though the lower pharynx is sometimes the seat of its production. It indicates a catarrhal affection of those parts.

HOARSENESS is a rough, harsh, grating quality of the voice that is heard under certain diseased conditions of the larynx and its muscular apparatus. When we hear a hoarse voice we may know that something is interfering with the normal action of the voice-producing machinery, preventing an harmonious rhythmical action in the parts. A growth may prevent the approximation of the vocal bands. Inflammation may thicken the whole mucous membrane, or the vocal bands themselves, or it may prevent those muscles from properly working, that control the position and tension of the vocal bands. Ulceration in the larynx may destroy more or less of the vocal apparatus, and thus bring about the trouble. Paralysis may also produce hoarseness.

Loss of Voice, or Aphonia, is usually ·due to paralysis of the laryngeal muscles, and this may be produced by inflammation, or by some trouble in the nerves which produce motion in the muscles. Of course extensive destruction of the larynx from any cause is followed by more or less loss of voice.

Painful Swallowing may be caused by pressure on inflamed and swollen parts during the act, or it may be due to ulcerated, raw surfaces being rubbed by the passing bolus of food.

Sense of the Presence of a Foreign Body may be caused by growths, presence of abnormal secretion, swelling, and excoriated surfaces that have been produced by rough food, bones, etc., scraping the mucous membrane.

Shortness of Breath may be due to inflammatory swelling partly closing the larynx, or a laryngeal growth may more or less prevent air from freely passing, or there may be a spasm of the muscles that bring the vocal bands together, or it may result from a paralysis of the muscles that open the glottis or laryngeal aperture ; but more frequently this symptom will be found to be due to disease of the bronchial tubes, lungs, or heart.

Sore-Throat is a painful sensation, produced by pressure on the end filaments of the nerves of the mucous membrane of the throat, by the swelling of that membrane from inflammation. Less frequently growths, such as cancer, exert the pressure. This symptom is most frequently confined to the lower pharynx where there is much motion, and where the act of swallowing increases the pressure on the tender nerves. Where there is much swelling, as in inflammations of the tonsils, the pain is very severe.

THE PRODUCTIVE CAUSES OF NASAL AND THROAT DISEASES.

TAKING cold is probably the most frequent cause of disease in the upper air-tract. This " taking cold " is the effect of exposures to extremes of temperature, which result in disturbances in the circulation of the blood, through mechanical and nervous influences. The normal temperature of the body is about 98° F., and its functions are interfered with more or less in proportion as that degree of heat is increased or diminished. Although exposures to excessive temperatures may act in different ways to bring about disease, as the effects are nearly identical, the process is generally spoken of as taking or catching cold.

The following are among the ways of " catching cold." A person may breathe air so cold that it acts as an irritant to the

mucous membrane of the air-tract ; this is
especially the case if the air is also damp.
Great cold may deprive the mucous membrane of so much of its vitality, that it is
not able to withstand the usual effect of the
blood-pressure of the general circulation.
A strong wind may blow into the nose, and
prove to be over-stimulating to the mucous
membrane.   If the whole body, especially
when the individual is overheated or per-
spiring, is unduly exposed to cold, there
will follow a general state of chill and de-
pression.   A reaction follows this state, and
it is apt to be an *over-reaction* which is peculiarly liable to affect in its excitement the
weak parts of the body; so, if the upper
air-tract happens to be the weak spot, it
will result in an inflammation of its mucous
membrane.   Again, a cold current of air
may strike one part of the body, unduly
cooling it.   The impression thus made may
be conveyed by the nervous system to certain nerve-centres, and thence may be reflected to the nose and throat, bringing
about an inflammatory excitement.   The
cooling of one part of the body may drive

out blood from that part into the weaker part, and thus start up inflammation.

These are the most frequent ways of taking cold. A less frequent method is the result of breathing too hot air, as one would be apt to do when employed over a stove, thus overheating the mucous membrane, partly depriving it of its vitality. This paralyzes the muscular tissue controlling the supply of blood in the blood-vessels, which furnish too great a blood supply to the part, and thus starts the inflammatory process. It is proper to state here that the taking of most colds is due to an improper regulation in the amount and distribution of the clothing worn. The fault may be in the fact that the whole body may be insufficiently clad, or it may be that a part of the body only, as the head or the feet, is not properly protected. Thin shoes, by causing cold or wet feet, have made numberless human beings miserable invalids. The next most frequent direct cause of throat and nasal affections is the inhalation of irritating matters in the form of dusts, vapors, or gases. Of course the atmosphere is always contaminated with floating impurities, and it is only when the impurities are in excess, or too irritating for the mucous surfaces which they come in contact with, that they become noxious. Among these impurities are the dust of the street, those produced in grinding and other pursuits, especially in tobacco factories, smoke, soot, chemical vapors, etc.

The lining membranes of the air-tracts of individuals differ in their sensibility to the same and different irritants. Thus, the well-known hay fever, which is a catarrh of the nasal tract and connecting mucous surfaces, is caused by floating plant pollen in the air ; it being quite harmless to the great majority of individuals, while it is the cause of disease in the hay-fever patient; and not only that, but some persons are affected by one kind of pollen, while others are affected by that of quite a different plant. The presence of a diseased condition in one part of the upper air-tract may be the cause of trouble in another; for example, nasal catarrh may cause laryngitis.

Again, those diseases that interfere with the proper circulation of the blood, such as of the heart and kidneys, may cause and keep up throat disorders. Inflammatory catarrhal attacks weaken the parts and predispose them to renewed diseased action. General constitutional weakness and delicacy of tissue predispose the individual to these affections.

Insufficient or improper nourishment, debilitating habits, residence in intemperate climates and unhygienic dwellings and surroundings, all have their effect on the causation of these troubles. Breathing foul air is a very prominent factor as a cause of nasal and throat disease, and in preventing their cure.

Locality is often the source of the trouble. It may be that the general locality is unsuited to the best hygienic needs of the individual, or some local source of dampness or impurity in the immediate vicinity of the dwelling may be at fault. Deprivation of sunlight may so depress the general physical health as to be the predisposing cause. The poisons of infectious diseases, the presence of foreign bodies in the air-tract, abuse of function, and functional disuse, especially breathing through the mouth instead of the nose, are also causes of the diseases under consideration.

THE DOMESTIC TREATMENT OF NASAL AND THROAT DISORDERS.

THE most successful treatment, in a domestic way, of the diseases under discussion, is such as will be preventive in its action. If the general health-status be maintained at a high level, the air-tract will participate in that good condition, and will be able to resist causes of disease that would otherwise bring about these disorders.

Proper food, regularity of habit, sufficient clothing, especially of the feet, plenty of muscular and out-of-door exercise, proper ventilation and heating of the family residence—and this means the breathing of pure air in-doors, free from dust and other impurities—are among the requirements of living up to a good hygienic standard. In the family it should be an aim to avoid undue exposure to those influences that cause these troubles, but yet efforts must also be

made to inure sensitive persons to a certain amount of exposure ; and among the
best means of doing this is the adoption of
a regular habit of cold sponge bathing, and
heating by means of the open-grate fire.
Sleeping-rooms should be kept well venti-
lated and tolerably cool, say from 50° to
60° in winter, and the terrible, elevated
temperatures of our furnace-heated homes
should be avoided. If there is an open
fire to sit by and warm one's self at, the
average general temperature of the house
need not be over 60°, except for great
invalids and the very weak and aged,
or in case of actual disease, where an elevated temperature may prove beneficial for
the case in hand. It is much better to
wear more clothing than to breathe air in
the house that is very much warmer than
the out-of-door atmosphere.

The ordinary *mild acute attacks* of the
upper air-tract have a tendency to quick
self-recovery if the patient be only protected from adverse conditions. Thus, if a
person with an ordinary attack of acute
"cold in the head," "sore-throat," or

" hoarseness," will remain quietly reclining and covered on a sofa or bed in an apartment moderately warm, eat a moderate, mild, unstimulating diet, and keep the intestines freely open, he will be surrounded by conditions favorable to a quick recovery. In case of sore-throat, ice may be melted in the mouth, or ice-water, with or without the addition of a mild astringent, may be taken in the mouth and allowed to bathe the inflamed parts. It is an important principle in the treatment of acute inflammations, that rest be given to the part inflamed ; so, if the larynx is the seat of trouble, talking, singing, etc., will increase the trouble. Acting upon the same principle, swallowing should be avoided as much as possible in attacks of sore-throat ; and frequent, forcible blowing of the nose, and breathing even an ordinarily irritating atmosphere, must not be done when a " cold in the head " is present.

SEVERE ACUTE ATTACKS should be treated only under the care of an intelligent physician.

CHRONIC nose and throat troubles usually need the attention of a competent physician. At least his assistance should be sought for, to point out the nature of the trouble and to suggest the outline of the treatment. In most cases this treatment can only be efficiently carried out by the trained surgeon, but most patients can assist in the cure by partial treatment at

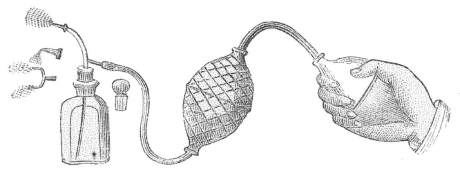

Fig. 10.

home. There is a large class of cases where regular cleansing of the nasal passages aud vault of the pharynx is an important and even necessary procedure. The cleansing fluid may need to be bland or stimulating as the particular case requires. It may sometimes be efficiently applied by snuffing it into the nose from the palm of the hand, but it is more desirable to possess a spray-producer to do

the cleansing with, constructed upon the
principle of the instrument represented in
fig 10. In the incurable cases of fetid catarrh,
such an instrument should be an adjunct of

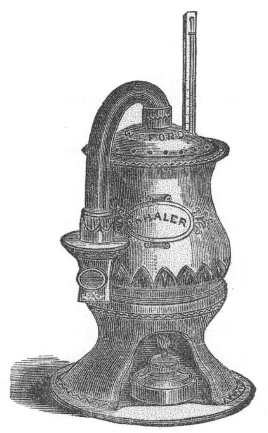

Fig. 11.

every toilet-stand, for, as in this condition
the nose cannot clean itself, the patient
should clean out his nasal cavities with as
much regularity as he would clean his
teeth or any other part of his body. In many

cases of throat trouble, the patient receives benefit from taking medicated inhalations at home. These can be taken from a regularly constructed inhaler, such as is shown in fig. 11 ; or, what is nearly as good, a pint of boiling water can be placed in a pitcher of convenient size, the medicament added, and the nose and mouth applied to the top of the pitcher, while a towel is held to the interstices between the face and pitcher so as to confine the steam, which is breathed into the throat for some minutes.

Sometimes a steam atomizer, shown in fig. 12, is very desirable to use. Of course

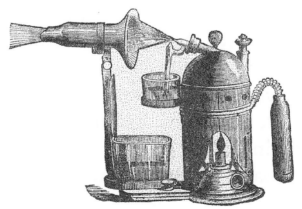

Fig. 12.

the various medical substances used in the inhalations should be indicated by a physician for the peculiar condition present.

THE immense improvement made
during late years in the treatment
of the class of disorders under discussion, has been greatly due to, and stim-
ulated by, the discovery and adoption
of the rather simple instrument known
as the LARYNGOSCOPE. The essential
part of this instrument is a small mirror
of a size fitted to the throat to be examined, attached to a long, slender han-
dle that allows the mirror to be held at
various angles at the back of the throat.
See fig. 13. This procedure enables the
operator to look around the corners, so to
speak, of the throat ; and after some practice, in overcoming the practical difficulties
of the examination, the observer can see
reflected in the small mirror almost all the
internal parts of the throat and the region

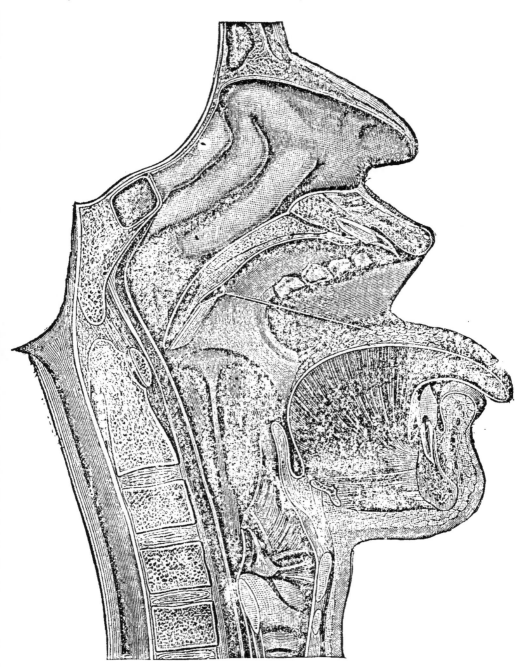

Fig. 13 shows the laryngoscopic mirror in position for viewing the larynx.

back of the nasal passages. The front parts of the nasal passages are inspected directly through the nostrils, which are dilated for that purpose with a proper instrument. Throat mirrors are represented in fig. 14. An essential to the working of the laryngoscope is a ray of intense light properly directed onto the throat mirror or into the parts to be examined. To attain this end the most convenient method is to use an artificial source of light, located at the side of the patient's head, which light is condensed and thrown on a perforated concave mirror attached to the forehead of the operator, and thence reflected through the open mouth onto the throat mirror as it is held in position ; or, if the front of the nose is under examination, the light is

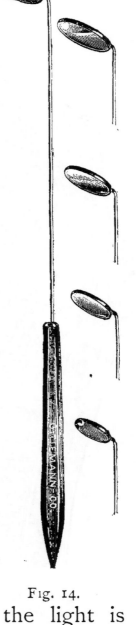

Fig. 14.

directed into the nostrils.   Fig. 15 represents.

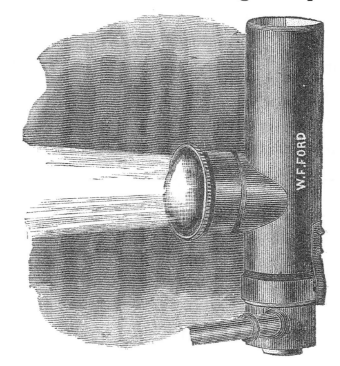

Fig. 15.

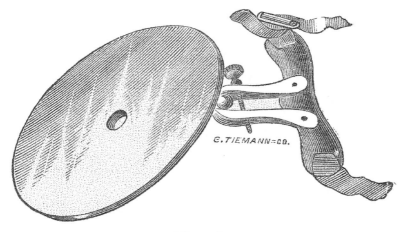

Fig. 16.

the light condenser most frequently used,

and fig. 16 the forehead mirror, through the perforation of which the operator gazes with the eye nearest the source of light, the other eye being uncovered, but shielded from the light by the rim of the mirror.

Fig. 17 shows the relative positions taken by the patient and the operator in the examination of the larynx by artificial light. Most of the lower pharynx can be examined without the throat mirror, the tongue being merely depressed with a tongue spatulum.

Having made the physical examination by the important means of sight, perhaps aided by feeling with the finger-tip, or various probes, and having the patient's history of his troubles, and the symptoms connected therewith, the experienced physician is enabled to arrive at a diagnosis of the case. This necessary and important preliminary being attended to, what can the surgeon do for the relief of the patient?

His treatment may be hygienic, constitutional, and local. Sometimes one method of treatment is sufficient; while

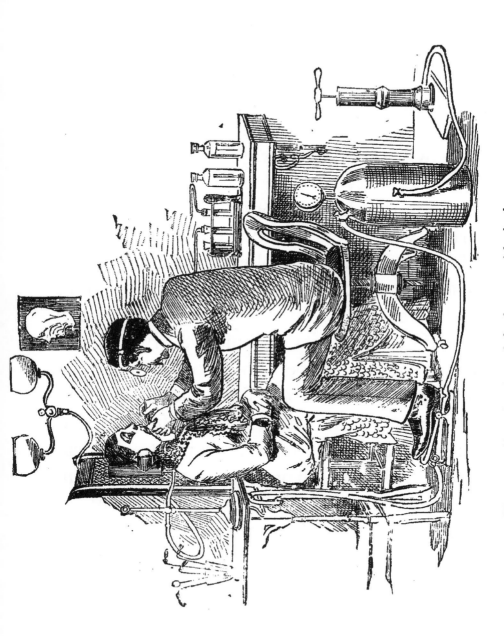

Fig. 17.—Examination of the larynx with the laryngoscope.

again, all are necessary. Frequently a mere pointing out of some infraction of hygienic living, and the correction of the same, will be all that is necessary to insure a cure. In some cases, only a very energetic course of internal medication will meet the exigencies of the case. The majority of cases coming under the care of the laryngologist are most appropriately and beneficially treated by a course of local medicinal applications made to the diseased structures—this course being more or less extended, according to the nature of the affection, or its chronicity. For example, a sudden hyperæmic condition of the larynx, causing a considerable amount of suffering to the patient, may often be entirely relieved by one appropriate application ; while old chronic cases, such as laryngitis, or post-nasal catarrh, can only be promised cure after a long and tedious course of treatment, very trying to the perseverance of the patient. It may be some compensation for such tedious cases to consider that, if they were not submitting to treatment, their difficulty would persist in-

definitely ; or, what is more probable, become progressively worse. The value of
making medicinal applications locally to
diseased structures of the body is so im-
mensely superior to the old method of internal medication that there can hardly be
instituted a comparison. As an example :
with the improved methods of to-day it is
possible to make applications to the trachea
and larger bronchial tubes, usually the seat
of bronchitis, and accomplish as much in
one day toward curing troubles in this part
of the body as could be done in four days
by giving medicines internally, besides
avoiding injury to the stomach and other
tissues of the body.

Of course the more strictly surgical
procedures are necessary in treating some
of the affections under consideration, such
as removal of the tonsils, enlarged mucous
glands, amputation of the uvula, etc., but
the majority of cases do not need such
rigorous treatment. Among the indica-
tions to be fulfilled in making local applications to the air-tract are the following :
1st, To CLEAN THE PARTS. 2d, To DISIN-

FECT. 3d, To PRODUCE A SEDATIVE ACTION. 4th, To RELIEVE PAIN. 5th, To AFFORD AN EMOLLIENT OR PROTECTIVE EFFECT. 6th, To CONSTRINGE THE PARTS, ESPECIALLY THE BLOOD-VESSELS. 7th, To STIMULATE THE PARTS. 8th, To PRODUCE AN ALTERATIVE EFFECT OR CHANGE IN THE ACTION. 9th, To RECOVER LOST FUNCTIONAL ABILITY. 10th, To DESTROY OR REMOVE REDUNDANT TISSUES. Medicinal applications are best made to the upper air-tract in the form of atomized sprays, produced through the agency of compressed air. Fig. 19 represents the usual compressed air-receiver, pump, and spray tube used for the purpose. Differently arranged tube-tips allow the operator to direct the sprays from different points into the various cavities. Sometimes the application is best made in the form of a powder, applied with an insufflator. Fig. 20 represents an insufflator that is operated by the air-pressure produced with a rubber hand-ball.

This is very convenient for personal application by the patient, and in the case of small children, who are apt to object to a

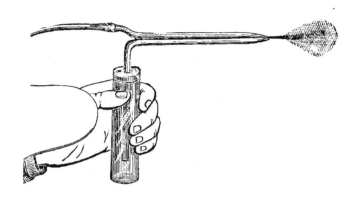

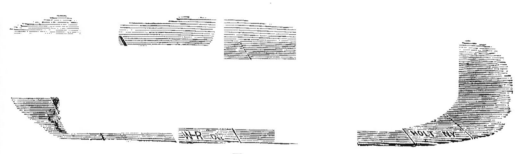

Fig. 19.

wet spray. Reference has already been
made to inhalations in the preceding chap-

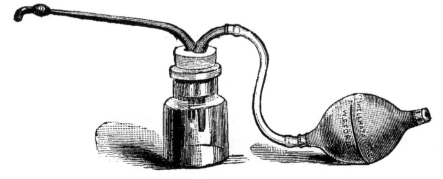

Fig. 20.

ter. Direct contact of medicated solutions by brushes, such as are shown in fig. 21, or by cotton pledgets wound on a probe, or by the solid drug fused on a proper instrument, are also methods of application. To produce the effects desired, the surgeon has open to his use the whole realm of chemical and pharmaceutical preparations, and a very long list of such substances are thus employed, many of them producing substantially the same effect. No two cases are entirely the same, and to produce the best result do not necessarily require identical treatment, nor does the patient require the same treatment at all times, it be-

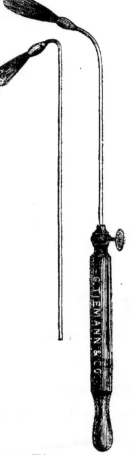

Fig. 21.

ing a matter of good judgment on the surgeon's part, at each sitting of the patient as to what remedies and measures are best fitted for the condition then present. Electricity has proved to be a remedial agent of such efficiency in treating certain of the diseased conditions under consideration, that mention of it should not be omitted. In its various forms it is used to effect removals of diseased tissue, and in re-establishing functional ability. In some hysterical cases its action is seemingly miraculous, one application of electricity to the larynx sometimes being sufficient to restore voice to a patient who has been voiceless for months or years.

ND - #0159 - 130622 - C0 - 229/152/5 - PB - 9780282687045 - Gloss Lamination